# the INSOMNIA Pack

*for when sleep is but a dream*

CHRISTINE FALVEY

# Contents

# *Contents*

*I have not slept one wink.*

William Shakespeare — *Cymbeline*

# Introduction

## What is sleep? What is insomnia?

*We tend to take sleep for granted until we don't get it. Then, when we experience the effects of loss of sleep, ouch! Does it hurt! Particularly when this goes on and on, night after weary day. The name for this unfortunate state of affairs, a prolonged inability to sleep, is insomnia.*

*Why is insomnia so terrible? Answer: because sleep is the only time in our daily lives when both body and mind, each in their own way, are in deep, refreshing rest.*

*That recuperation occurs in stages. Most physically beneficial is the deep or delta sleep period. This is followed by REM (Rapid Eye Movement) sleep, the sleep in which we dream. Light sleep, the kind believed to be the most beneficial to the intellect and the psyche, is the final, finishing stage.*

*I had followed the green, luminous course of the second hand and the minute hand and the hour hand of the bedside clock through their circles and semi-circles, every night for seven nights, without missing a second, or a minute, or an hour.*

Sylvia Plath — *The Bell Jar*

Lack of sleep is a health hazard. Exhausted insomniacs are at greater risk than sound sleepers of accidents at work and at home or traveling between the two. The chronically sleepless tend to become unhealthily overweight from eating to replace the energy they're not getting from healthy sleep. When we sleep we produce more interleukin 1, a chemical that stimulates our immune systems. When we don't sleep well and regularly, we strain our immune systems, our defense against disease.

*O polish'd perturbation! golden care!*
*That keep'st the ports of slumber open wide*
*To many a watchful night!*

William Shakespeare — *Henry IV,* Part 2

# WORRYING ABOUT SLEEPLESSNESS WON'T HELP

UNLESS WORRY LEADS YOU TO ACTION. AS ALL INSOMNIACS KNOW, YOU CAN'T NAG YOURSELF TO SLEEP! IRONICALLY, OFTEN THE FIRST ACTION RECOMMENDED IS TO STOP WORRYING. COLD COMFORT TO INSOMNIACS DESPERATE FOR SLEEP, AND EASIER SAID THAN DONE, OF COURSE, BUT WORTH A TRY AND MORE EASILY DONE IF THERE'S SOMETHING PRODUCTIVE YOU CAN DO TO HELP YOURSELF.

BUT IF YOU'RE AN INSOMNIAC, BE CONSOLED. YOU ARE NOT ALONE. YOU ARE ONE OF SEVERAL MILLION PEOPLE WHO FREQUENTLY FIND IT HARD TO GET A GOOD NIGHT'S SLEEP.

*Sleep appears to be rather addictive. Many find that they cannot do without it and will go to great lengths to ensure its possession. Such people have been known to neglect home, hearth, and even publishers' deadlines in the crazed pursuit of their objective*

Fran Lebowitz — *Metropolitan Life*

Some find it hard to fall asleep, but sleep like logs when they finally do. Others say that they are asleep as soon as their heads hit their pillows, yet, an hour or so later, they're awake, a pattern that will repeat throughout the night. Others complain that they never get back to sleep until five minutes before they're due to wake.

Some suffer insomnia for years, others for shorter periods of time, usually during passages of extreme stress on and off throughout their lives.

These days, sleeping pills are the last resort in terms of treatment. Reputable practitioners of Western medicine are loath to prescribe them because of the well-documented side effects, ranging from headaches to addiction.

Moreover, there's so much you can do to help yourself using natural methods, with or without the assistance of your personal healthcare practitioner. Even those suffering such serious sleep disorders as sleep apnea, nocturnal myoclonus, narcolepsy and the weariness that is symptomatic of some forms of depression can look forward to gaining some measure of relaxation by natural methods.

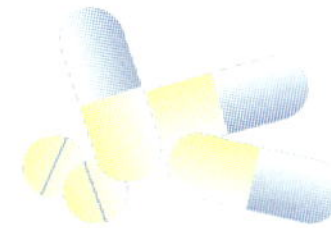

*I did not sleep. I never do when I am over-happy, over-unhappy, or in bed with a strange man.*

Edna O'Brien — *The Love Object*

# *Famous Insomniacs*

THOMAS ALVA EDISON

*Dear Thomas invented the lightbulb like the one in your bedside lamp by which you might be reading this. Thomas is a shiningly bad example to all insomniacs because he firmly believed sleep to be a waste of time, and worked as hard to reduce his need for sleep as you try to fulfil yours.*

RUDYARD KIPLING

*The sun never set for him any more than he believed it would set on his beloved British Empire.*

FRIEDRICH WILHELM NIETZSCHE

*Nietschze was a wildly influential insomniac whose indomitable sense of humor enabled him to reflect in his* Human, All Too Human *that, "The thought of suicide is a great consolation; by means of it one gets successfully through many a bad night." Note that he recommended nothing more drastic than contemplation.*

NAPOLEON BONAPARTE

*Most people think that the great French general simply said, "Not tonight, Josephine." Actually, he said, "Not tonight, Josephine, I've a pile of despatches from the front to read, just as many awaiting reply, and much strategic thinking to do. In other words, ma cherie, I've a lot of worrying rather than a lot of living to do. I'll be awake all night doing it and certainly cannot contemplate anything that might distract me from my obsession with developing heroic bags under my eyes." Delusions of grandeur, megalomania, ambition, call it what you will, it was all to no avail come Waterloo.*

## *American Presidents who suffered insomnia*

Franklin Delano Roosevelt

Harry S. Truman

Dwight D. Eisenhower

John Fitzgerald Kennedy

Lyndon Baines Johnson

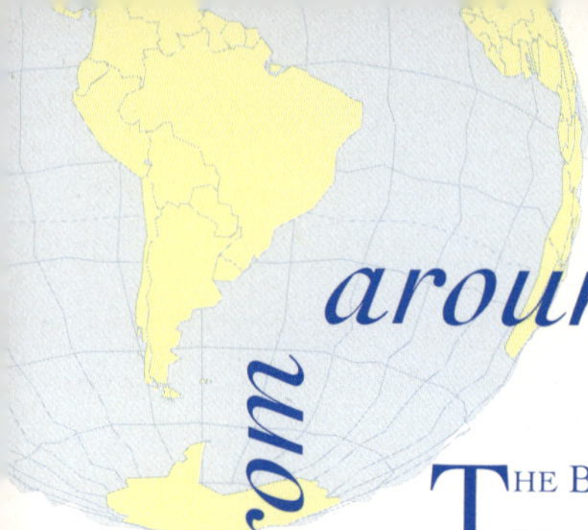

# *Insomnia Cures from around the World*

The Burmese recommend nibbling on pollen cakes at night to induce sound sleep.

Pueblo Indians consume large quantities of mushrooms as a late night snack to be sure of a sound and lasting sleep until well after sunrise.

Warm milk with or without an egg, and a dash of honey, brandy, or both, is a bedtime remedy the length and breadth of England.

Generations of Chinese families follow the tradition of sipping ginseng tea for tranquillity as they review and then farewell the preceding day.

ROMANY GIPSIES SHARE A BREW PRODUCED BY BOILING A LARGE HEAD OF LETTUCE IN A POT OF SALTED WATER, AND WATCH THE FLAMES OF THEIR CAMPFIRES SETTLE BEFORE RETIRING.

FROM THE INDIAN SUB-CONTINENT COMES THE AYURVEDIC PRESCRIPTION OF A CUP OF SWEETENED AND WARMED MILK LACED WITH A PINCH OR TWO TO YOUR TASTE OF CARDAMOM (*ELETTARIA CARDAMOMUM*) WITH NUTMEG (*MYRISTICA FRAGRANS*) OR A FEW THREADS OF PRECIOUS SAFFRON (THE DRIED, GOLDEN STIGMA OF THE AUTUMN-BLOOMING PURPLE *CROCUS SATIVUS*).

SLEEP

HOW MUCH SLEEP DO YOU NEED? YOU. NOT YOUR MOTHER, YOUR SISTER OR BROTHER, YOUR BEST FRIEND, YOUR LOVER. SOME OF US CAN'T GET BY ON THE MUCH-QUOTED EIGHT HOURS'

# *Sleep Management*

SLEEP IN TWENTY-FOUR. AND SOME FIND THEY PERFORM AT PEAK LEVELS INTELLECTUALLY, EMOTIONALLY AND PHYSICALLY WITH FOUR HOURS' SLEEP, WHILE OTHERS NEED SIX HOURS' SLUMBER AT MOST.

SLEEP

*The Student sleepes six Howres, the Traueller seuen; the Workeman eight, and all Laizie Bodies sleepe nine Howres and more.*

Wodroephe — *Spared Hours of Soldier*

*Six hours sleep for a man, seven for a woman and eight for a fool.*

18th-century proverb —
A favorite of England's George III

*Is there not a proverb that a man requires six hours sleep, a woman seven, a child eight and only a fool more: If this be true, thousands of great men were, and are, fools.*

The Spectator

*John Wesley ... considered that five hours sleep was enough for him or any man.*

J.H. Friswell — *Gentle Life*

*One houres sleepe before midnight is worth three after.*

G. Herbert — *Outlandish Proverbs*

# A Sleep Journal

Strangely enough, many of us don't know exactly what's good for us in the way of sleep. To clarify your sleep needs, record the actual hours you spend sleeping over a period of one or two weeks. Some find a small tape recorder near their pillows is easier to work with than pencil and paper.

Note the time you go to bed and the time you actually snuggle down to sleep, as well as your natural awakening time. If you're an on-again-off-again sleeper, keep note of those periods, too. And don't neglect to count any catnaps you take during the day.

*And so to bed.*
Samuel Pepys — *Diary*

*I haven't been to sleep for over a year. That's why I go to bed early. One needs more rest if one doesn't sleep.*

Evelyn Waugh — *Decline and Fall*

YOUR NOTETAKING SHOULD ALSO INCLUDE A DETAILED LIST OF TYPES AND QUANTITIES OF THE FOOD AND DRINK YOU HAVE CONSUMED THROUGHOUT THE DAY AS WELL AS WITHIN AN HOUR OR TWO OF BEDTIME.

RECORD ANYTHING AND EVERYTHING YOU THINK MIGHT BE PERTINENT: CHANGES IN THE WEATHER, SLEEP DISTURBERS SUCH AS SQUEALING TIRES, HOWLING CATS, PARTYGOERS, SNORING PARTNERS, SWINGING GATES OR RATTLING WINDOWS.

*He hath slept well that remembers not he hath slept ill.*

17th-century proverb

# *Stress*

## Relieving stress in your life is often the way to relieve your insomnia.

*Canst thou, O partial sleep, give thy repose*
*To the wet sea-boy in an hour so rude;*
*And in the calmest and most stillest night,*
*With all appliances and means to boot,*
*Deny it to a king: Then, happy low, lie down!*
*Uneasy lies the head that wears a crown.*

William Shakespeare — *Henry IV,* Part 2

Don't dismiss the deceptively minor stresses in your life. They can join up to create a seething mass of anxiety that would daunt the staunchest character.

So tend to the small fry first, the ones that seem to be nibbling only at the edges of your life; given half a chance, they will eat your sleeping hours away.

YOU MIGHT NEED TO KEEP A STRESS JOURNAL – SIMULTANEOUSLY WITH YOUR SLEEP JOURNAL IF YOU LIKE, PARTICULARLY IF YOU'RE AWARE THAT YOUR DREAMS ARE TO SOME EXTENT MIRRORS OF WHAT'S GETTING UNDER YOUR SKIN DURING YOUR WAKING HOURS.

IF YOUR DREAMS OR NIGHTMARES ARE WAKING YOU, MAKE A NOTE OF THEM FOR SUBSEQUENT ANALYSIS. OUR DREAMS ARE OFTEN THE KEY TO THE UNRESOLVED STRESS TROUBLING OUR SLEEP.

GET INTO THE WAY OF CHECKING ON EXACTLY WHAT IT IS YOU'RE FEELING, PHYSICALLY AND EMOTIONALLY. ARE YOU TIRED, OR MORE DEPRESSED THAN TIRED? TIRED, OR MORE WORRIED THAN TIRED? TIRED, OR VAGUELY ANXIOUS? ARE YOU MORE HUNGRY OR THIRSTY THAN TIRED? OR VICE VERSA?

*I pray you, let none of your people stir me: I have an exposition of sleep come upon me.*

William Shakespeare —
*A Midsummer Night's Dream*

# STRESSBUSTER TECHNIQUES

*The thing to do is to get an opera score and read that.*

Marilyn Horne — American diva

**DO SOMETHING NEW.** If you're in the habit of sleeping badly, chances are your life's stuck in a miserable rut of some kind or other. Break out of that rut by doing something different and pleasurable. The idea is to throw your habits, all of them, into turmoil. Trust yourself to keep the good ones and not miss the life- and soul-destroying ones such as insomnia.

Leave your bed if you must to go and look at the moon, home of the Sea of Tranquillity. The Sea of Tranquillity. Repeat it over and over to yourself, to the moon itself, to all the night creatures (yes, the cockroaches, too) prowling and scurrying in their other-world peak hours.

Drop into an executive giftstore. Stress-busting toys for big boys and girls are their specialty. Take your pick from all sorts of battery-operated, time-wasting, mesmerizing gizmos, including slam-dunk wastebaskets and punching balls for your desk or bedside.

*A gentleman sleeps at his work. That's what work's for. Why do you think they have the SILENCE notices in the library? So as not to disturb me in my little nook behind the biography shelves.*

Alan Ayckbourn —
*Round and Round the Garden*

Pack up your troubles. Use your imagination to stow them someplace they can't escape until you say so. Put them in the biggest envelope in the world, a steamer trunk that would sink the Titanic, the vault at Fort Knox.

*Try thinking of love, or something.*
*Amor vincit insomnia.*

Christopher Fry — *A Sleep of Prisoners*

Be contrary. Stop telling yourself: I must go to sleep, I must go to sleep, I must go to sleep. Instead, snuggle down into your bed while promising yourself: I will not sleep, I will not so much as shut one eye.

# *Bedtime Rituals*

A big no-no for insomniacs is irregular hours. To regulate your sleeping patterns, try setting an alarm after dinner to remind you that it's time to go to bed, and don't get caught in front of the television set. Reset the alarm to wake you at your chosen time the next morning. The trick is to go to bed at, say, 10pm, and get up at the same time, anywhere between 6 and 7am, say 6.30am, no matter what. No matter if you didn't doze until 4am.

*Susan: … I watch far too much television,*
*if you can call that relaxing.*
*Bill: Oh, yes. Rather. Best sleeping draught there is.*

Alan Ayckbourn – *Woman in Mind*

Some people claim that television is the best soporific they know. If you're determined to bring good sleep back to your life, avoid watching anything too upbeat, dramatic or scary – and certainly not within an hour of your planned bedtime.

Similarly, all work, whether housekeeping chores or files from the office, should be tucked away at least an hour before you plan to tuck yourself in.

Plan to give yourself at least a week, maybe two or three, during which you eat a light evening meal before about 7pm and take a post-prandial stroll or other moderate exercise for fifteen minutes or so.

Give yourself plenty of time to complete your individual getting-ready-for-bed routine, which may include an aromatherapy bath or massage, a slowly sipped cup of herbal tea, teeth-cleaning, bed-warming, fiddling with blinds and curtains, and putting clothes away and preparing the morrow's before you crawl between your sheets.

While you're following this program, the only naps you should take are those you deliberately factor into your timetable — and then only one per day, after lunch, and absolutely for no longer than thirty minutes.

*What hath night to do with sleep?*

John Milton — *Comus*

NOR SHOULD YOU SLEEP IN ON WEEKENDS. OTHERWISE, COME SUNDAY NIGHT YOU MIGHT BE OVERWHELMED BY THE SLEEP-DEFEATING COMBINATION OF A WELL-RESTED BODY AND A MIND KEYED UP TO COPE WITH THE FORTHCOMING MONDAY TO FRIDAY.

*But sleep had been taking a vacation from her; as if she were a pariah, it visited her too infrequently, and then only out of unavoidable duty.*

Octavia Waldo — *Roman Spring*

THE TIME WILL COME WHEN YOU WON'T NEED THOSE AFTER-DINNER, LIGHTS-OUT ALARM BELLS. YOUR CLEVER LITTLE BODY-CLOCK WILL HAVE FALLEN INTO THE RHYTHM OF THINGS AND HAVE YOU TANGOING OFF TO BED ON YOUR TIPPY-TOES, DELIGHTED AT THE PROSPECT OF SLUMBER THAT'S AS EASILY ACHIEVED AS IT'S BEEN HARD WON.

*How many thousands of my poorest subjects*
*Are at this hour asleep! O sleep, O gentle sleep,*
*Nature's soft nurse, how have I frighted thee,*
*That thou no more wilt weigh my eyelids down*
*And steep my senses in forgetfulness?*

William Shakespeare —
*Henry IV,* Part 2

THAT SAID, IF YOU CAN'T SEEM TO STOP YOUR MIND DARTING OFF IN ALL SORTS OF TROUBLING AND RANDOM DIRECTIONS, OR IF YOU HAVE A BAD CASE OF THE BEDTIME FIDGETS, YOU SHOULD RECOGNIZE THAT THIS IS SOMETIMES PART OF THE VERY NATURAL PROCESS OF RELEASE — FROM A STATE OF INTENSE BUT NECESSARILY CONTROLLED ANXIETY AND AGITATION DURING THE DAY. THINK OF IT AS A BUFFETING TIDE AGAINST WHICH YOU CAN'T SWIM. TRUST IT TO CARRY YOU TO A GOOD PLACE, EVENTUALLY, AND GO WITH THE FLOW.

HAVENS ARE HIGHLY PERSONAL THINGS. FOR SOME A BEDROOM HAVEN FEATURES A BED WITH CRISP LINEN SHEETS METICULOUSLY FOLDED BACK. FOR OTHERS, A SHAMBLES IS HEAVEN.

AND FOR SOME OF US, A CHANGE IS AS GOOD AS A HOLIDAY. IF YOU'RE OBSESSIVE ABOUT FOLDING YOUR BEDCOVER, YOU MIGHT FLING YOUR CARES AWAY IF YOU WERE TO FLING

# *Creating a Haven in your Bedroom*

THE QUILT TO THE FLOOR BEFORE THROWING YOURSELF ONTO YOUR MATTRESS. OR, IF YOUR BEDROOM LOOKS LIKE A BOMB HIT IT, WHAT ABOUT A TIDYING-UP BLITZ?

ONE NIGHT WHEN YOU JUST CAN'T SLEEP, WHY NOT MAKE A LIST OF WHAT CONSTITUTES YOUR PERFECT SLEEP-SPACE?

YOUR BED: LARGE OR SMALL, SOFT OR HARD. UNDERLAYS: ELECTRIC BLANKETS OR SHEEPSKIN RUGS. SHEETS: SILK OR SATIN, COTTON OR LINEN, WASH 'N' WEAR? COVERS: BLANKETS OR QUILTS, ONE OR MANY?

*"It would make anyone go to sleep, that bedstead would, whether they wanted to or not."*
*"I should think," said Sam,*
*"Poppies was nothing to it."*

Charles Dickens — *Pickwick Papers*

YOUR ROOM: BLACK AS PITCH OR BATHED IN MOONLIGHT? NOISES OUTSIDE: A WORRY OR A COMFORT? TOO HOT? TOO COLD? AIR-CONDITIONED OR TEMPERATURE CONTROLLED BY MOTHER NATURE?

ACCESSORIES: DO YOU LIKE BEDSIDE LAMPS THAT BARELY GLOW, OR DO YOU LIKE A LIGHT TO READ BY WITHOUT STRAIN? DO YOU HAVE A DECENT RADIO, ONE THAT DOESN'T SPLATTER AND CRACKLE AS THE COW JUMPS OVER THE MOON, ONE WITH SNOOZE AND ALARM BUTTONS THAT ALLOW YOU TO DRIFT OFF AND TO WAKE FROM SLEEP WITHOUT HAVING TO REACH FOR THE CONTROLS? DO YOU HAVE A CASSETTE OR CD PLAYER SO YOU CAN CHOOSE YOUR OWN BEDTIME MUSIC?

THERE MAY BE SOME THINGS YOU CAN DO NOTHING WHATSOEVER ABOUT, BUT THERE ARE BOUND TO BE SOME SLEEP-INDUCING CHANGES YOU CAN MAKE.

For instance, new blinds and curtains might be beyond your budget, but sleeping masks are not a luxury item — certainly not for an insomniac.

Think about babying yourself by listening to a tape of lullabies. Even those with lyrics in unfamiliar languages share universally soothing qualities. Many music stores and alternative therapy stores stock large ranges of music or sounds known to soothe and tranquillize, and also music for meditation.

Don't like the feeling of masks — the elastic worries your ears and drills a channel in the back of your skull? Insomniacs are expert at converting minor irritations like this into major, life-threatening traumas. OK, then use a sleep sachet. These soft dumplings of comfort, filled with scented, sleepytime herbs, rest light as a feather across your frantic eyes.

Ever thought about earplugs? Big problems sometimes require only small solutions.

# Positive Thinking

WHETHER, LIKE OGDEN NASH'S TOMATO SAUCE COMING OUT OF A BOTTLE, YOU'RE ONE WHO NEEDS SLEEP EITHER A LITTLE OR QUITE A LOTTLE, THE EXPERTS AGREE: DON'T TRY TO SLEEP UNLESS YOU'RE FEELING SLEEPY.

NOR SHOULD YOU UNDERESTIMATE THE BENEFIT YOU GET SIMPLY FROM RESTING IN YOUR BED. REST IS A GOOD THING. MAYBE IT'S NOT AS GOOD AS THE SLEEP YOU NEED, OR THINK YOU DO, BUT, GIVEN THAT YOU CAN'T SLEEP, MAKE THE MOST OF YOUR REST. DON'T SPOIL PERFECTLY GOOD REST BY FRETTING BECAUSE YOU'RE NOT ASLEEP.

For the stuff you can't change, can't resolve, can't even begin to understand, get philosophical. Shrug. Go on, actually shrug. It *is* possible to live in the question without driving for the answer.

# *Relaxation*

*Men who are unhappy,*
*like men who sleep badly,*
*are always proud of the fact.*

Bertrand Russell —
*The Conquest of Happiness*

RELAX

# *Breathing to Sleep*

TAKE A DEEP BREATH.
THEN ANOTHER.
THEN ANOTHER.

When you're abed, it's easy. Wriggle down into the bed so you can raise your arms to rest behind your head, palms facing upward. Have a good stretch, pointing your toes ahead, your fingertips behind you. Breathe in through your nose, allowing your abdomen to expand as you fill your lungs. Exhale as slowly as you can through your mouth, sensing as you do the exit of tension from your body and then from your mind.

## *Meditation*

Breathing can also be used as a meditation technique. Focus on the effect of each breath on that tiny area of your face below your nostrils and above your upper lip. After a few minutes you will relax, your breathing becoming easy and gentle.

You can also meditate simply by choosing a word or sound that appeals to you, and silently repeating it to yourself. Try to synchronize each repetition of the word as you breathe out. Welcome any thoughts that drift into your mind, but just let them drift on by to somewhere else. Don't try to solve any of your problems right now. Resume repeating your mantra. If you persist, you will become aware that your mind is not only a place of disquiet but also a place of quiet.

## *Progressive Muscle Relaxation*

This is one of the simplest and most effective techniques to prepare mind and body for sleep.

Lie comfortably in bed, and, starting with the top of your head, tense and relax each part of you. Crinkle your face, clench your teeth. Relax.

Flex and unflex your arm muscles, your shoulder, neck and back muscles. Clench and unclench your hands. Tense and release your stomach, buttock, thigh and calf muscles. Curl and uncurl your toes.

You could then move straight to a subtle, non-stretching variation of deep breathing. Inhale through your nose and, as you exhale through your mouth, envisage the release of all the tension remaining in your body. Continue until you become comfortable with your breathing and settle into a relaxing rhythm.

Relax

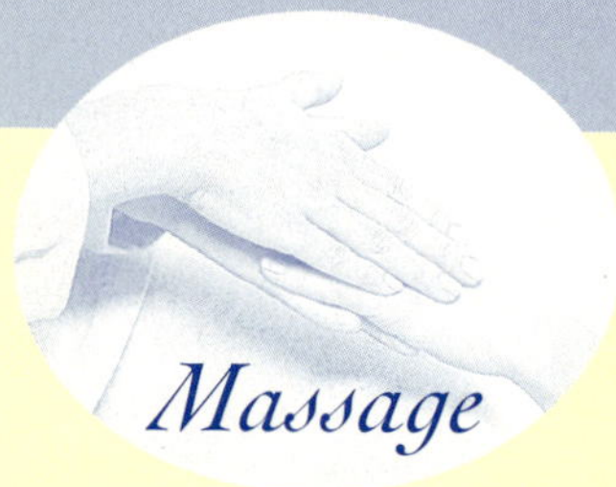

# Massage

How about some self-massage? How about massage from a sympathetic friend? How about a mutual massage with your lover? Mmmmm! And ... Zzzzz!

Use one of the sleep-promoting essential oil mixtures (see pages 55–61) to massage your hands and feet, popular repositories for storing much of the excess stress and tension that are the enemies of sleep.

To massage your hands, begin by using the fingers of one hand to stroke the other gently from wrist to fingertips. Then use the forefinger and thumb of one hand to rub firmly between the fingers and knuckles of the other. Next, take each finger and pull from base to tip in a gentle, corkscrew movement. Now use the thumb of one hand to massage the palm of the other. Finish by using each hand to smooth the other gently from fingertips to wrist.

To massage your feet, start by spreading a little oil over your left foot and resting it on your right thigh. Now hold your left foot with your left hand, and use the knuckles of your right hand to massage the entire sole. Firmly massage the ball of the foot —the padded part behind your toes — with both thumbs. Squeeze and wriggle your toes. Arch your foot. Stretch it, toes pointing upward. Pinch the tip of each toe. Finally, with your left foot on the ground, stroke from the toes with both hands to encircle your ankles, repeating this final, soothing gesture as often as you like. Repeat the whole process for your right foot.

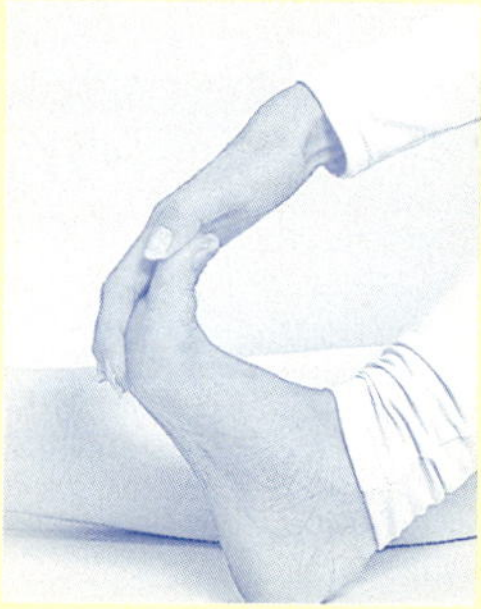

To massage your left shoulder, move the palm and fingers of your right hand in a counterclockwise stroke, beginning at the edge of your shoulder and then going toward your back and on to the side of your neck, down over the edge of your collarbone and back to your shoulder's edge. Repeat three to five times. Next, push with your fingers into the muscles on and behind your shoulder, maintaining on-the-spot pressure on the ones that are tender and moving them in tiny circles, clockwise and counterclockwise, until they ease. Then repeat the first, shoulder-massaging stroke. Now, with your fingertips making circular movements, move your hand up the side of your neck from your shoulder to behind your left ear. Finish with another shoulder massage. Repeat the entire procedure for the benefit of your right shoulder and the right side of your neck.

# *Exercise*

We know exercise makes you look good and live a longer or at least healthier life. But how many of us know that it can help improve our sleeping patterns by making us feel good? Not simply virtuous, nor the endorphin-induced buzz known as a runner's high. But happy, relaxed, calm and on-top-of-things. And you don't have to run a marathon, even work up a sweat, to reduce your sleep-ruining anxiety. All you need to do is: get rhythm — and take it easy.

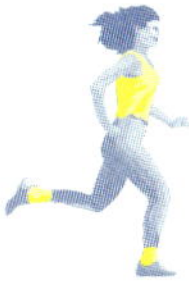

For it's *rhythmic* aerobic exercise, such as a brisk but comfortable walk, an easy, smoothly swinging run, a relaxed bicycle ride or a few gentle laps of a swimming pool (backstroke or breast stroke alone or in combination — your favorite stroke is the best for you) that reduces anxiety.

Half an hour or so of moderate and rhythmic exercise will reward you with a calming effect that should last for about two hours, enough to carry many of us into the sleep we need.

Insomniacs seeking aerobic fitness should plan their vigorous exercise from early to mid-morning or from late afternoon to early evening before dinner. They certainly shouldn't gain a super-trim body at the expense of their sense of mental well-being by giving up any of their early-morning light sleep.

# *Food and Drink*

## What to Have, What to Avoid

*For his sleep was aery light,*
*from pure digestion bred.*

John Milton — *Paradise Lost*

*Skipping breakfast and lunch and then devouring a big dinner can be disastrous for insomniacs. Effectively, you're asking your poor old metabolism to work overtime — all through the night in fact, although everyone knows metabolisms need their beauty sleep.*

*Perhaps you've heard yourself saying something like, "I'm too tired to eat. I just want to go to bed." Chances are that's exactly when you need something light but nutritious, something that's quick and simple to prepare.*

*A piece of fruit, a handful of dried fruit or nuts or both, a glass of milk. Come on! Force yourself to stagger to the kitchen! A minor midnight raid might be all you need to set you up for hours of blissful shuteye.*

The ideal meal plan for insomniacs is three light but nutritious meals daily, with healthy snacks mid-morning and mid-afternoon and something soothing at bedtime.

Tea, coffee, caffeine-loaded cola drinks, the demon alcohol. All are stimulants and theoretically not a good idea as pre-bedtime drinks.

But sometimes, a little of what you fancy does you good. Better the moderate approach than a grimly obsessive one. If you're a sherry-drinking insomniac, you might enjoy a glass of Manzanilla sherry, which is flavored with the mildly sedative chamomile herb.

*Recent research indicates that carbohydrates are calm-you-down food, not just because they make you feel sated, but also because they raise the level of the amino acid tryptophan in the brain. There it becomes the neurotransmitter serotonin, which triggers a chemical message of the feel-good kind.*

*The onset of this relaxation response occurs about forty-five minutes after eating complex carbohydrates (bread, cereal, pasta, vegetables, popcorn and rice cakes), but only about five minutes after eating simple sugars such as the refined sugar widely used as a sweetener, or those in fruit juices.*

*If you mix carbohydrate with protein, though, the effect is quite different, protein being a stimulant.*

*Celery, cloves, cumin, fennel, ginger, sage and parsley — all are also serotonin stimulators producing a natural tranquillity.*

*Onions contain the relaxant quercetin. So, if your sleeping partner doesn't mind ...*

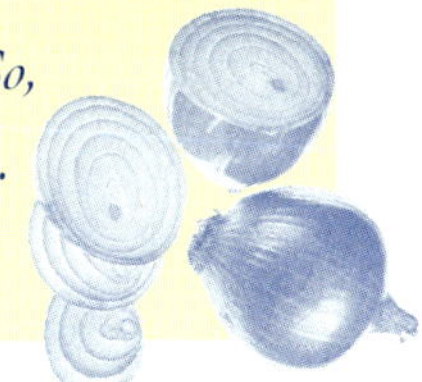

# *Herbs to Help*

## Teas — Inhalations
## Sleep Pillows — Bath Sachets

*Many herbal teas are now available in teabag form. If not, a basic recipe is to pour about 7 fl oz (200 ml) boiling water onto 1 teaspoon dried herbs, or 2 teaspoons fresh herbs. Pour through a strainer and allow to cool a little, so that you can sip the tea slowly.*

*Chamomile flowers (whether from the German plant,* Matricaria chamomilla, *or the common or so-called Roman variety known as* Chamaemelum nobile *or* Anthemis nobilis*) make a gently soothing tea.*

Red clover, readily available in teabags for city-types deprived of the pleasure of gathering their own sweet-smelling, sweet-tasting flower heads, is as good a relaxant as it is a taste sensation and is popular with children, too.

V is for valerian (*Valerian officinalis*), the ground root of which is a super-sleepmaker that does not interfere with the REM state or produce any lingering, post-sleep drowsiness. Unfortunately, many people find valerian tea unpalatable. A few suitable additives can solve this difficulty. To 2 teaspoons valerian add 1 teaspoon lemon juice or cider vinegar or other fruit-based vinegar, plus 3 teaspoons honey.

Ever noticed a cat luxuriating in catmint (*Nepata cataria*) before taking a catnap in the sun? This herb's pretty pink-to-mauve flowers and tiny leaves are used to make a tea that will relax your nerves and muscles as a precursor to sleep.

Another herbal tea recommended for insomnia is Asian skullcap (*Scutellaria baikalensis*). It is favored by Chinese physicians as a tranquillizer and a sedative. If preferred drink it with honey and lemon.

The flower from the bergamot plant (*Monarda didyma*) is a delightful soporific, too. It is similar in scent and anxiety-reducing properties to the oil extracted from the rind of the small fruit of the bergamot tree (*Citrus bergamia*) that flavors Earl Grey tea.

## Other herbal treasures for your tea chest include:

Comforting melissa or lemon balm (*Melissa officinalis*)

Relaxing rosemary (*Rosemary officinalis*)

Vervain or verbena (*Verbena officinalis*), which assists in the easing of nervous tension and depression

Soothing lime or linden flowers (known as either *Tilia cordata* or *Tilia europaea*)

Sweet, wild marjoram (*Origanum vulgare*), or equally sweet but also spicy knotted marjoram (*Origanum marjorana*) to counter nightmares or fearful feelings

A mild limeflower tea is a gentle relaxant that most children find acceptable, particularly if it is sweetened with honey.

A tea made with equal quantities of limeflowers, melissa and aged and dried hops (*Humulus lupulus*) will also help insomnia.

You could use this mixture, or the time-honored limeflowers alone, to stuff a small, soft sleep pillow for your head or a larger sachet to scent your bedsheets.

The recipe for the following sachet mixture comes from a manual for 17th-century European noblewomen:

*Take dried rose leaves, hops, powder of mints, powder of cloves ... put all together in a bag and take to bed with you to cause you to sleep — and 'tis good to smell unto at other times.*

Make a bath bag just as you would a sleep sachet. Fill it with a handful of vervain, bergamot leaves, rosemary or melissa. To release the scent of the herbs, swing the bag under your hot-water tap while your bathtub fills, and from time to time, while you're soaking in your bathtub, swirl the sachet through the water to freshen the fragrance.

The healing practice of aromatherapy, using the essential oils extracted from particular plants, goes back about five thousand years and has been used by the ancient Indian practitioners of Ayurveda (Sanskrit for "the science of healthy life"), and the ancient Egyptians, Greeks, Romans and Chinese.

# Essential Oils for Sleep

Modern scientific investigations have reinforced the reputation of essential oils of effecting complex, natural chemical interventions and interactions to restore a healthy balance to our minds and bodies.

Being such a nurturing, pampering, sensual approach to what ails us, aromatherapy is made for most insomniacs, whether we're full-blown neurotics or just amateurs, going through a bad patch at the office, worrying about our mortgages, driven to temporary distraction by a formidably adolescent child or pining for a lover lost or far away.

Pharmacies, supermarkets, health food stores, your friendly naturopath – all are sources of supplies of the essential and carrier oils and ready-made combinations for special purposes, including the relief of insomnia.

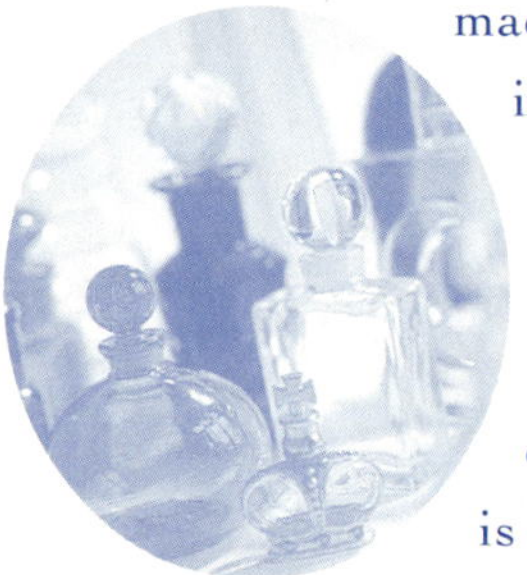

Aromatherapy oil suppliers also stock aromatherapy equipment such as spray bottles and vaporizers (either electric, or those where the oil and water mixture is heated and aromatized by burning a small candle).

You probably have some aromatherapy equipment at home already, in the form of your bathtub and your kitchen bowls. Fill them with warm water, and add a few drops of your chosen mix of essential oils. Inhale or soak yourself – simultaneously, if you're in the bathtub – toward tranquillity. Desirable drowsiness is not far behind.

You can also sprinkle your essential oils directly onto your pillow, or tuck a fragrant facial tissue or handkerchief into the pocket or sleeve of your nightshirt.

Scent your scarf, sit-up-and-snooze collar or sleeping mask when you're an overnight passenger on bus, train or plane. Close your eyes and bring to mind fields of lavender releasing a blissful aroma into the heat haze of a summer's day.

Many experienced aromatherapists would give lavender oil pride of place in treating insomnia and some of its causes and symptoms: anxiety, tension, agitation, fear, restlessness, grief and depression.

LAVENDER: *Lavanduala vera, Lavendula officinalis* OR *Lavendula angustifolia* — take your pick of the many names by which the true pinky-purple lavender is known.

FOR A SUSTAINED, BENEFICIAL SLEEP, EXPERIMENT WITH THE FOLLOWING BLENDS OF LAVENDER MIXED WITH OTHER ESSENTIAL OILS IN YOUR VAPORIZER:

*4 drops lavender plus 2 drops bergamot (from the peel of the baby fruits of the bergamot orange tree* Citrus bergamia*), an oil with anti-depressant, calming, balancing, sedative qualities.*

*2 drops lavender plus 4 drops either Roman chamomile (*Chamaemelum nobile *or* Anthemis nobilis*) or German chamomile (*Matricaria chamomilla*).*

*4 drops lavender plus 2 drops soothing, tranquillizing neroli bigaradia (from the blossom of the bitter orange tree,* Citrus aurantium amara*) or 2 drops sweet orange oil (*Citrus sinensis*).*

*Babies, too, respond well to a chamomile and lavender mixture. If your poor wee bairn seems to be getting off to a rotten start as one of life's bad sleepers or is in the habit of waking self and household every few hours, place a facial tissue scented with two drops of each between the bedsheets about an hour before bedtime. When it's time for bed, slide the little one in and the scented tissue out. Sing a lullaby or two. Leave a dim nightlight to comfort the baby should it stir, and to allow you to check on it during the night without disturbing its sleep.*

*A single drop each of lavender and chamomile in a baby's bath is also recommended for a calming effect.*

AND NEVER DISCOUNT THE RESTORATIVE PROPERTIES, FOR OLDER CHILDREN AND ADULTS, OF A WARM BATH TO WHICH HAS BEEN ADDED ONE OR OTHER OF THESE LAVENDER BLENDS:

*2 drops lavender with 2 drops chamomile*

*1 drop lavender with 1 drop calming, relaxing frankincense (the resin of the small Arabian tree,* Boswellia carteri*) and 2 drops neroli*

*4 drops lavender with 4 drops marjoram (*Origanum *or* Marjorana hortensis*, sweet marjoram, the "joy of the mountain") and 2 drops orange (from the rind of the bitter orange tree,* Citrus aurantium*)*

*3 drops lavender with 3 drops neroli*

*2 drops lavender with 2 drops neroli and 2 drops chamomile*

*3 drops lavender with 3 drops marjoram*

OR YOU COULD SIMPLY ADD 5 OR 6 DROPS OF ONE OF THESE OILS TO YOUR BATH.

*The way to health is to have an aromatic bath and scented massage every day.*

Hippocrates

OTHER ESSENTIAL OILS KNOWN TO INDUCE RESTFUL SLEEP AND SUITABLE FOR BATH OR VAPORIZER INCLUDE:

GERANIUM (*PELARGONIUM GRAVEOLENS*)

LIMEFLOWER OR LINDEN (*TILIA VULGARUS OR CITRUS AURANTIFOLIA*)

MELISSA OR LEMON BALM (*MELISSA OFFICINALIS*)

ROSE (*ROSA DAMASCENA*)

VALERIAN (*VALERIAN OFFICINALIS*)

VETIVER OR VETIVERT (*VETIVERIA ZIZANOIDES*)

YLANG YLANG (*CANANGA ODORATA*)

Mothers-to-be beset by insomnia will benefit particularly from the combination of lavender, rose and chamomile in bath or vaporizer.

They will also take comfort from 3 drops ylang ylang added to a bedside vaporizer or a bowl of hot water for an inhalation, or sprinkled directly onto pillow or pajamas.

Ayurvedic practitioners recommend using cold pressed sesame or coconut oil to gently massage the two major marmas or touch points for sleep — one in the middle of the forehead, the other just below the navel — with light, clockwise strokes.

FOR A SLEEPYTIME MASSAGE SOLUTION, ADD UP TO 20 PERCENT BY VOLUME OF YOUR FAVORITE ESSENTIAL OIL TO A BASE CARRIER OIL SUCH AS SWEET ALMOND OR SAFFLOWER OIL.

CHOOSE FROM LAVENDER, LEMON BALM, LIMEFLOWER, PEIITGRAIN (NEROLI'S DELICATE COUSIN, MADE FROM THE LEAVES AND SHOOTS OF THE BITTER ORANGE TREE, *CITRUS AURANTIUM AMARA*), GERANIUM, VETIVER OR YLANG YLANG.

SOME SLEEP-INDUCING BLENDS ARE:

- *Bergamot with neroli, lavender or geranium*
- *Chamomile, rose and lavender, good during pregnancy*
- *Frankincense with sweet orange and neroli*
- *Ylang ylang with vetiver, rose or neroli*

MANY MEDITATORS FIND THAT BURNING ESSENTIAL OILS ENHANCES THEIR CONTEMPLATION.
THREE OF THE MOST POPULAR OILS FOR THIS ARE FRANKINCENSE, NEROLI AND ROSEMARY.

# Professional Help

## When Home Remedies Aren't Enough

MOST PEOPLE EXPERIENCE SLEEPLESS NIGHTS WHEN THEY HIT A ROUGH PATCH IN LIFE. IF THEY'RE LUCKY, THE MIND AND BODY WILL SOON, QUITE UNAIDED, RECOVER THEIR PERSONAL, ESSENTIAL EQUILIBRIUM BETWEEN SLEEPING AND WAKING HOURS.

OTHERS HAVE NO SUCH LUCK. SO IF YOUR INSOMNIA IS THE PERSISTENT, LINGERING, DRIVE-YOU-CRAZY VARIETY WHICH ALL THE SELF-HELP YOU CAN MUSTER HAS EASED ONLY A MITE, THE SMART THING IS TO SEEK PROFESSIONAL HELP. AND IF YOUR INSOMNIA IS ACCOMPANIED BY FEELINGS OF SADNESS, INEXPLICABLE TEARFULNESS, LACK OF CONCENTRATION, WEIGHT LOSS OR GAIN OR EVEN THE SLIGHTEST HINT OF A DEATH WISH, SEEK PROFESSIONAL GUIDANCE IMMEDIATELY.

SOME SERIOUS SLEEP DISORDERS ARE VIRTUALLY IMPOSSIBLE TO SELF-DIAGNOSE ACCURATELY. FOR INSTANCE, SLEEP APNEA SUFFERERS ARE TYPICALLY UNAWARE OF THE PRECISE NUMBER OF TIMES THEY STIR SLIGHTLY BUT SUFFICIENTLY TO DISRUPT THEIR SLEEP AND EVENTUALLY PRODUCE SERIOUS, EVEN FATAL CONSEQUENCES. ALLERGIES, TOO, CAN BE TRICKY THINGS TO TRACK DOWN ON YOUR OWN.

YOUR HEALTHCARE PRACTITIONER SHOULD BE VERY IMPRESSED WITH THE ARSENAL OF COMMONSENSE REMEDIES YOU'VE DIPPED INTO AND ANY INSIGHTS YOU'VE GAINED INTO YOUR INSOMNIA. HE OR SHE SHOULD BE ONLY TO HAPPY FOR YOU TO CONTINUE TO USE THESE NATURAL REMEDIES AS YOU WORK TOGETHER TO FIND A GREATER MEASURE OF RELIEF.

*I shall sleep like a top.*
William Davenant — *The Rivals*

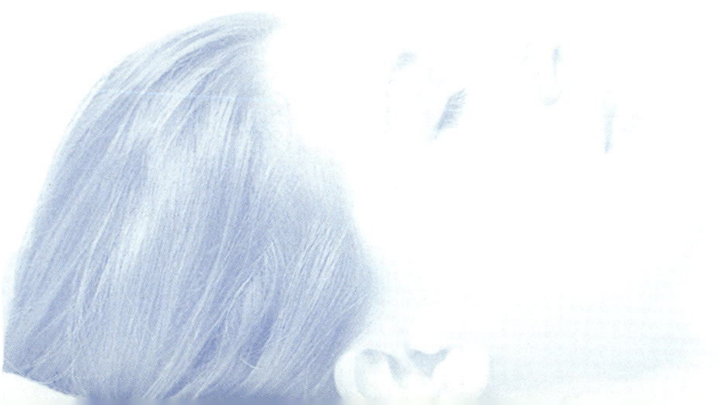

This book presents information and material about home remedies. This book is intended to supplement, and not replace, treatment by a physician or other licensed medical practitioner. Consult your health care provider before adopting any of the treatments described herein. The adoption and application of the material offered in this book is at the reader's discretion and sole responsibility. The author and publisher of this book are not responsible in any manner whatsoever for any injury that may occur indirectly or directly from the use of this book.

First published in The United States of America in 1997 by Journey Editions, an imprint of Charles E. Tuttle Co., Inc. of Rutland, Vermont, and Tokyo, Japan, with editorial offices at 153 Milk Street, Boston, Massachusetts, 02109.

Published in conjunction with Lansdowne Publishing Pty Ltd
Sydney, Australia


ISBN 1-885203-42-X

Designer: Sylvie Abecassis
Cover design concept: Liz Seymour
Set in Cochin on QuarkExpress

10 9 8 7 6 5 4 3 2 1

Printed in Hong Kong